The
Third
Component

Adam Schaeuble

ISBN-10: 1535034793
ISBN-13: 978-1535034791

This book is dedicated to my wife and kids.
Thank you for helping me write the best chapters of my life!

CONTENTS

The Final Day of the Old Me

Part One: Setting Yourself Up For A Successful Transformation

Part Two: Going From Goal Setting to Goal Achieving

Part Three: Fitness and Nutrition Fundamentals

Part Four: Save Time, Money, and Effort by Avoiding Common Mistakes

Part Five: Finding Your Healthy Lifestyle Balance

About The Author

Taking Action With Adam and His Team

Client Testimonials

THE FINAL DAY OF THE OLD ME

I know I'm supposed to be "Mr. Positive Fitness Dude" and everything but when I see that Facebook post I can't help but think "another one bites the dust". You know the post I'm talking about..."Just finished Day 1 of my Couch To 5K Program....So Excited!". I see at least one of these a day, yet I have NEVER EVER seen a post that says "I just finished my entire Couch to 5K program! Wippeee!"

Have you ever felt like you have tried EVERY freakin diet out there?

Have you ever purchased a year gym membership only to end up using it for about six days total?

Have you ever felt like you wanted to take some action to become healthier but you just couldn't figure out where the heck to start?

The problem is that goal setting is a lot of fun and very motivational indeed. Planning for and then starting something new brings a lot of excitement and energy to our lives. This is especially true when it comes to health and fitness. We humans are *awesome* at "planning", "getting ready for", and "starting" things like a new diet, fitness regimen, or going to a new fitness facility.

I got my start in the fitness industry by working the front desk at a locally owned fitness center called The Iron Pit Gym. I started in the summer time and I got the hang of things pretty quickly. I would sit there all day, chat about protein powder, and then sign a few people up in between. Around mid December the owners pulled me aside for a pep talk to prepare me for what would happen on January 1st. I fondly remember this as the "New Years Resolutioneers Are Coming" talk. I was warned that business would pick WAAAAAY up with everyone making their New Year's Resolution to finally make this *their year* to get in shape. So January 1st hit and the flood gates opened. I signed people up for memberships all day long and not just short term stuff.....these people were in it for the long haul because *this was their year*. I sold more 12 month memberships in one day than I had all summer long! The facility was packed with newbies! Fast forward to January 7th.....one week into the deal and at least half of the newbies would be gone. Fast forward another week and 90% of the newbies were done. It blew my freakin mind! At the time I barely had enough money to get by and I was living off of spare protein powder that the owners gave me because it tasted so bad that no one else wanted it (root beer float flavor....delicious!). I couldn't fathom that someone would make that type of a financial commitment and then give it their all for a whole TWO WEEKS and then quit!

I quickly came to realize that the entire "I am getting ready for something and I have serious goals" process is fun and it makes us *feel* like we've been productive, but what have we really accomplished? The answer is a big fat NOTHING. You have taken an important step, but it is just the first step in the overall process.

With this book I want to help you as the reader, as my new *student*, to first be able to understand my unique processes and then be able to implement them. As we start this new student/coach relationship you need to understand that I have an abundance of energy and reading this book may feel a little bit like taking a drink of water from a fire hose at close distance! I have not included any fluff in this book because I don't have any patience for that. I have some concepts and processes that I 100% know will be game changers for you and I am personally driven to show you how to implement them effectively. Take your time and make notes as you read. When the action steps pop up, take a second and actually work through them. Reading this book should not be a passive experience for you. I want you to take action!

We know that goal setting is the right way to start things off, but it is the goal *achieving* that we are really after.....and that is going to take some work so let's get started!

People will start a transformation for many different reasons. There is usually a moment where they get smacked over the head by the old "frying pan of life". This is a jarring moment when a person realizes that there must be a change of momentum. This is a huge moment because you have officially taken your blindfold off. Too many people will just continue to go with the flow of life.......even though they know deep down that they aren't maxing out their life's potential.

My moment came in early July of 2007. When I think back about my life, there are only a handful of moments that I specifically remember in detail and this is definitely one of those moments. I was standing in the middle of the grocery store with my credit card in hand. I weighed around 330lbs at the time and I was heading down a bad road with my long term health. I had been a strength coach for the last four years and I was unhappy with where my career was. I was mainly training athletes......high school kids that is. I was surrounded by bratty teenagers day in and day out. Now there were a FEW good ones in there that I really enjoyed working with, but for the most part I was a 300lb muscle bound baby sitter! Although my health was not great my social life was showing some promise. By some miracle... I was able to gain the attention of a female while I was at the Iron Pit Gym working out and we had started a serious relationship. This was definitely the best part of my life. Then she dropped a bombshell on me that she was going to move up to Indianapolis (about an hour away) to pursue her doctoral degree. So let's go back to the grocery store.......I'm standing there with my credit card in hand. I've already racked up about $40,000 of credit card debt at this point and I'm not even sure that I have enough room on the card to pay for my groceries. This was the *exact* moment in time that I realized that I had become a CRAP MAGNET. The bad stuff was sticking to me like glue and I couldn't get away from it. The negativity would consume me day in and day out and it was taking it's toll on my life. We have all been to the old Crap Magnet Hotel but I was engaging in an extended stay and I realized that I had to find a way out.

Now I wasn't the only one that saw my amazing crap magnetism. My friends were very much aware. I think some of them started to avoid me just to ensure that they "didn't get any on them". I did have a friend that tried to help me out. He had given me a DVD called *The Secret* a few weeks prior to my M.C.M.R (Moment of Crap Magnet Realization). I took it home for a few days, just to be nice, and then I brought it back and said "how awesome it was".......even though I didn't actually watch it. Then it happened AGAIN. Another friend brought me the DVD and insisted that I watch it. This time I let the DVD sit on top of the DVD player for a few weeks. I was much too busy watching re-runs of the *World's Strongest Man* to be bothered with this positivity hocus pocus! Now that I think back on all of this, I realize how close I came to being stuck where I was as a full time CRAP MAGNET. After my rock bottom moment at the grocery store I went home and made an important decision. I had attended a conference earlier in my career and I remembered a man saying "For things to change YOU must change and for things to get better YOU must get better." I decided that this was my time to change. I noticed that DVD sitting there when I got home so I decided to pop that in and see what this "positive thinking" stuff was all about. My life has dramatically improved with each *second* that has passed since that very moment. I'm hoping that you are experiencing a similar effect.....right about NOW.

July 8th, 2007

I was ON FIRE after finally realizing that I had to reverse all of this negative momentum and consciously make an effort to *get better.* After watching that DVD I started to immediately drink the positivity Kool-Aid on a daily basis. I felt like my eyes were opened and I had electricity running through my body. It is really amazing to think about how many missed opportunities there are when you are stuck in that negativity rut. It was like the lights got turned on in the room and I could see all the great things I had to take advantage of that had been right there in front of me all along! I had my first taste of personal development material with *The Secret* and I was craving more of the same. I started to read a new book every week and I decided to turn my car into The University of Positivity on wheels by only listening to personal development materials instead of music. I was downloading and purchasing anything I could get my hands on by authors like Tony Robbins, Robert Kiyosaki, Og Mandino, Stephen Covey, and Dale Carnegie.

I came to the point where I made the decision to plan out the life of my dreams. I called this my Lifestyle Rehabilitation Plan. I mapped out my life that I wanted to create for myself over the next five years. I chose five years because I figured that was a long enough time frame to get some substantial things done to overhaul my life. Now did I 100% believe that all of this stuff would actually come true.......not really but I thought that even if a few of these things happened I would be so much better off compared to my days as a CRAP MAGNET.

So I imagined myself pulling up to the "Drive Thru Window of Life" and I placed my order! I started off the process by making a list of goals that I wanted to achieve. It looked something like this:

- Lose 50 lbs (Funny side note....Every guy that weighs over 300lbs assumes that if *they could just get down to 275lbs* that they would be ripped......not so much.)
- Have ideal health stats including blood pressure, blood sugar, heart rate, cholesterol, and body fat %.
- Married with at least one child
- Have at least 10 employees on my team. Leveraging my talents by having other people help me out.
- Leverage my time by creating a business format where I can work with several people at once.
- Leverage my time by creating an online business.
- Have a studio of my own that is over 6,000 sq feet. (I have no idea why I picked this number but it just sounded about right to me.)
- Zero personal or business debt........living in abundance.
- Have a healthy balance between work, personal, and family time
- Enjoy my life on a daily basis

Next I transformed this list into my Lifestyle Rehabilitation Statement™. There were FIVE key rules:

1. Everything had to be written with a positive focus.
2. Everything had to be written in the present tense as if it were already true.
3. I had to really try to FEEL IT as I read it.
4. There had to be a set deadline. My deadline was July 8th, 2012 which was five years from the date I wrote my Lifestyle Rehabilitation Statement.

5. I had to commit to reading this statement *every damned day*, twice per day, until everything came true or the deadline passed.

Here is the result:

"It is July 8th, 2012. My life is incredible. Every day I wake up and realize that it is going to be a great day. I am healthy and fit with all of my health stats in the ideal ranges. I feel strong and I enjoy my workouts that have produced a low body fat level. My business is hugely successful. Team NGPT has great momentum as we provide services that not only produce great results but we have the ability to positively impact the lives of all of our clients. Our 6,000 sqft facility is in an excellent location and our clients love coming in for their workouts. I have a wonderful family that I love very much. I have a balanced schedule and I take advantage of my opportunities for work, personal, and family time. I live in abundance whether at work or at home and each day is better than the last one."

The next 12 months:

I believe that the ability to achieve goals is very much determined by our personal momentum. Over the next year my life went through a huge momentum shift. Depending on how bad things are it can take a lot of time and energy to really shift directions and that was the case for me......but I stuck with the plan. I read my Lifestyle Rehabilitation Statement every damned day, twice a day and I was feeling it! I was able to drop 50lbs, reduce my credit card debt to about half, and I got my personal relationship with my girlfriend (soon to be fiancé) figured out. The momentum was building for me big time! I decided that it was time to start going after some of the BIG goals so I sat down to make a battle plan. I looked over my original goals list and I asked myself "Which one of these would have the biggest impact on my life if it came true?". This is the goal that I chose: *Leverage my time by creating a business format where I can work with several people at once.* My thinking behind this choice was that if I could help more people achieve their goals it would have a trickle down impact on everything else I wanted to achieve myself.

Now the next step I took was a LIFE CHANGER. I will never forget this moment and I am so proud of myself for making the decision to just take a leap of faith and go for it. I made the decision that I had to take ONE action step towards this goal right away........like RIGHT NOW. I had recently started to attend some Thai Boxing classes at a local martial arts studio called Monroe County Martial Arts. I was really loving it and the owners of the studio were great people and ran a great business. I had an email that I had written out that I wanted to send to the co-owner Linda to propose an idea for a martial arts blend group fitness class. I wanted to use their studio to launch the concept and make it innovative and fun. I was really excited about it but I was scared to death to send that email to her so there it sat.....for several weeks in my drafts file. When it came down to it I knew that this was a big opportunity for me but I didn't have much self confidence at the time and I knew that a rejection could really derail my momentum. After accepting my own personal challenge to take immediate action I knew what had to be done. I immediately went to my drafts file, gave it one last proof read, and hit SEND.

July 15th, 2012………Five years (and 8 days!) later

When the alarm went off at 4:30am I knew this was a BIG day. I got up out of bed and kissed my wife on the forehead. I took a second to peek in at my son Henry before I walked out the door. As I drove in to work that day I thought about the last five years. I thought about reading that Lifestyle Rehabilitation Statement….every damned day…twice a day. I thought about how good it felt to pay off that last credit card. I thought about the day I proposed to Marissa, the day we got married, and the day our son Henry was born. I reflected on the positive impact that Team NGPT had on the lives of over 600 people in our local community. I thought about the thousands of pounds that had been lost through the program that I was lucky enough to create. I thought about how I had been able to lose over 100lbs personally and redefine my own idea of being in great shape. As I pulled into my parking spot at our brand new 8,000 sq foot studio I knew this was a special day. This was the day that I got to check off my last goal that I had set for myself five years ago. YES…I KNOW…I missed my deadline by a whole EIGHT DAYS! As I walked into the studio I greeted everyone that was there like I always do. I mingled with the crowd as we all talked about how exciting it was to have this new facility for the program to really flourish. In the back of my mind I just kept on thinking about how lucky I was that things fell into place for me to be able to completely change my life. Five years ago there had been no guarantees that any of this would have become reality. I was just a young man that was trying to get his life together. It freaks me out every time I think about those key moments in the beginning that helped me shift my momentum and then of course there was the email to Linda. That was the moment that my positive momentum went into overdrive. She fully supported me and my idea and the rest is history. All I needed was that ONE person that I really respected that supported my idea and that was the fuel that ignited my entrepreneurial FIRE for the next five years. So as we got ready to start our very first workout at the new facility I made my little speech and thanked everyone for helping me achieve the goals that I had set for myself and our program. I was really proud of myself for taking control of my personal situation, shifting my momentum, taking daily action in the correct direction, and ultimately knocking out and *achieving* every one of those five year goals that I had set for myself.

So what did I do next? I took some time to reflect and celebrate what I had accomplished and THEN I decided to go back to that Drive Through Window of Life again by resetting all new goals for myself..........which I read every damned day....twice a day! One of my new goals is to be able to leverage my time and energy and figure out new ways to help even MORE people including YOU. My key action step that is the equivalent of the "Linda Scott Email" is writing THIS book. You might be right where I was when I started. You may be the Mayor of Crap Magnet City! All I will ask of you is to believe in this process and take daily action. YOU and your goals are worth it. There is a reason that this book fell into your lap and I hope that one day you realize that this was a key moment in your life that sparked an amazing swing of positive momentum.

PART ONE:
SETTING YOURSELF UP FOR A SUCCESSFUL TRANSFORMATION

The most cost effective way to lose weight is to lose each pound only ONCE. For some people those will be hard words to read. We all know how hard it can be to lose weight. It is even harder, both mentally and physically, to re-lose weight after you have gained it back. In this part of the book we are going to focus on the strategic thinking steps that you need to mentally process before you truly are able to engage in an efficient and effective transformation.

The Amazing Results Formula

For those of you that fit into the category of "I've tried everything and I can't get the results I want!", this formula is going to be an eye opener! When I mention this magic formula to clients their ears always perk up as they prepare to receive some sort of super duper secret fat blasting exercise. So sometimes they are underwhelmed when I present the following:

$$(SNP + SER + ST) + (C/T) = AR$$

OR

(Solid Nutritional Program + Solid Exercise Regimen + Strategic Thinking) + (Consistency/Time) = Amazing Results

When people decide it is time to lose some weight they will most often attack either the first or second component individually by doing things like starting a diet or signing up for a gym membership. This is a critical mistake. When I first started doing personal training I had a few clients that were paying me top dollar to provide great workouts with my personal training services, but they had no interest in changing their nutrition so their results would be nonexistent. This scenario will lead to people quitting altogether because in their mind they are putting in all this hard work and not seeing any results. In reality, you just can't out work poor nutrition. There is also the scenario where people will only focus on a diet regimen and not add in any physical exercise at all. I feel like this is also a recipe for an early burn out because the results are going to be slow moving and oftentimes the nutrition component will be based off of a fad type of diet that isn't maintainable long term anyway. So a really great first step is to make sure that you are active with BOTH of the first two components of the formula at the same time.

The third component of *Strategic Thinking* is what this book is all about. People almost never think strategically about their health, nutrition, and fitness. I know top level business owners that have a killer structure in place for their business that involves all kinds of goal setting, monitoring, and accountability. Why not map out your health game plan in the exact same way? I think we all can admit that we, as human beings, kinda suck at the consistency over time component as well! It seems like as "the going gets tough" we just decide to take zero ownership over the situation and just try something else and hope that it might work.

How many of you out there have read a diet book and stuck with it for a whole two weeks or signed up for an eight week bootcamp only to attend the first week? We all like to dive into that "getting started" process but too often we never develop a specific game plan and we have no accountability structure to set us up for consistency. Once a client asked me to break down the importance level of nutrition and exercise when it comes to the overall transformation process. I came back with 10% nutrition, 10% exercise, and 80% strategic thinking. I don't think that was the response they expected!

I've had the privilege of being in the fitness industry since 2001 and I've been able to work with over 1,000 local clients (from my hometown of Bloomington, IN!) with our nutrition, exercise, and coaching programs. Between 2009 and 2015 our hometown clients lost over 35,000 LBS and I have definitely been able to see some patterns emerge. One pattern that has come to the forefront time and time again is how important the strategic thinking component is to the overall transformation process. By "strategic thinking" I don't mean the ability to sit and think the pounds away.....that would be pretty awesome though! I'm talking more about having your head in the game, understanding what could derail your transformation, knowing what you are getting into, being motivated, staying motivated, being accountable, and having a strategy in place at all times. Some of you may have tried MANY different exercise and nutrition programs in the past. Do an honest self evaluation as to why you stopped, switched, or quit that program.

If you are truly being honest you will come up with an answer that deals with the mental aspects of the transformation process:

- I got bored.
- I cheated too much on the diet.
- I couldn't maintain my motivation.
- It was too hard.
- I couldn't stay organized.
- Life just happened and I got off track.

The only two valid reasons to actually quit a program would be that you did everything 100% correctly and got no results or you sustained some kind of injury and had to stop. Anything else is going to be due to the mental component kicking in. This can be a hard pill to swallow for most of us. We will cover the topic of taking ownership over our situation a little bit later so just hang in there!

The main goal of this book is to help you put together the proper structure for your strategic thinking component so that you can stay focused and motivated, get the best possible results, and maintain those results over the long haul. We want to shorten your learning curve by applying each component of the Amazing Results Formula.

The mind is a powerful yet scary place and that is where most of our battles will be fought in a transformation. We are our own worst enemy at times, but the great news is that we can also use our minds to overcome many of the false limitations that we have for ourselves.

When someone comes to me and they are in bad physical condition I have to attack their bad habits with a vengeance. It has taken them years and years to build up and solidify those bad habits and I usually have a few months to try to totally reverse their momentum......now that's tough! That is also why not everyone makes it through to the other side.

I'm hoping that you to have an "Aha!" moment at some point as you read the information I am going to give you. Once that light bulb flips on and you become 100% mentally focused you will feel unstoppable and the physical transformation goals will be *achieved*. I truly believe that you can take the core principles that you will learn in this book and apply them to any fitness and nutrition regimen and get much better results in a shorter amount of time. The information you are about to read will help you fill in the gaps in the process in order to go from just starting a transformation to becoming *transformed*. Each and every one of us deserves to feel like we are in control of our health and feel that amazing personal momentum that comes along with it!

TAKING ACTION:

Throughout the book you will get a few prompts to start taking action. I recommend that you start a file on your computer or tablet and save your notes as you go through this book and do the action steps.

- <u>Action Step</u>: Review the Amazing Results Formula again. Think about each component and make notes on which components you feel like you have locked in really solid and which ones need improvement. We all have to start somewhere and this is where you will start to build your supporting framework for your transformation process. You will get some great ideas on how to improve each component throughout this book.....especially the Third Component!

The Transformation Timeline

The Transformation Timeline is a concept that I came up with after I realized that there were always three barriers (pain points) that people had to cross to get to a place where they could successfully maintain their results. To have an effective transformation process you need to understand where you are at in the transformation timeline at all times. It is also critical to learn what danger zones are preventing you from crossing to the next phase of the timeline.

The first barrier deals with being coachable. This pain point almost always occurs when someone is four to six weeks into their new transformation process. The key fork in the road at this pain point deals with how people react to being coached and held accountable. The people who fall out at this point will take any coaching/accountability as being judged or pressured. The people who pass the test realize that for things to change *they* must change their habits and the only way to get there is to be coached and be held accountable. The constant in the equation is the coaching and accountability. The variable is how you are going to view it.

You have to actively make that choice that you are going to give in to whatever program or fitness professional you are hiring to help you. This has to extend past the point of the initial transaction. Some people think that "Hey I paid them so that shows that I'm coachable!"…..not so much. The transaction is the easy part, the hard work begins right after that point. With our programs we plug our clients into a high accountability system where we require them to send daily reports to a coach. If they don't send those reports, the coach tracks them down. Our clients have to actively think about whether or not they will remain coachable during that initial phase of our program. Will they send that report or not and will they get it done daily?

Back when I first started my personal training business I had a client named Bill who was doing several sessions a week with me but refused to let me guide him along with his nutrition. In our first three years together he lost 30lbs....which is not too shabby. In year number four though, he decided to become 100% coachable and let me have control over his nutrition as well. He lost almost 40lbs in the next three *months*. So he lost 30lbs in three years being half way coachable and then 40lbs in three months by being 100% coachable. I think it is common for people to not want to give up 100% control like this. You just have to trust the expert that you have given your money to and give them an honest shot to perform the service that they have been hired to do! If you wanted to become fluent in a foreign language you wouldn't hire a tutor and listen to 50% of what they said because that just wouldn't work and it would be a huge waste of your time. The same rules should apply to your health and fitness!

The second barrier deals with solidifying your new healthy lifestyle. This pain point usually occurs after people have lost 10-25% of their bodyweight or they at least have seen some pretty major results. The key fork in the road at this pain point deals with the question "Am I really willing to commit to this new lifestyle?".

The people who stall out at this point will start to do a lot of projection or make excuses as to why they can't continue this new healthy lifestyle. When people fail to cross this barrier they will say things like "I'm getting bored." or "This isn't maintainable." The people who keep making progress will take ownership over this new lifestyle and realize all of the awesome benefits that come with it. At this pain point people realize that this whole transformation thing is going to be a challenge. The initial success was awesome and it may have even come easily for some, but now the grind starts and only the people that stay positive and accept this as "the new normal" will pass to the next stage.

I always listen for some key language as people talk about what they eat. If they talk about being on a "DIET" they are usually stuck at this pain point. If they talk about a "nutrition strategy" or say things like "THIS IS HOW I EAT!"....then they are on the right track. A *diet* is something that is temporary. Your goal should be to implement a sound nutritional strategy that results in a healthier way to eat and live for the long haul.

The critical mistake that people make at this point is that they think that "I've got this and I can do it on my own now!". This is when people start to mess with their routine and go a little rogue. In reality you have spent many years building up the bad habits that put you into less than optimal health and you've only been doing this new regimen for a few months at this point. Those bad habits still lurk close to the surface and we still need to keep our focus. This is the point where you have to really dial in with your program and work on making your new exercise and nutrition plan a routine habit and solidify this new healthy lifestyle.

The third barrier deals with creating a new self identity and purpose once you have reached most of your goals. This is especially important for people with large weight loss goals. We've had the privilege of helping several people lose over 100 pounds and with each one I was able to see this barrier appear. This pain point usually occurs when people are very close to hitting their weight loss goals or have been within that last 5%-10% of their goal range for about 6 months or more. The question of "what's my new purpose and/or identity?" comes to the forefront when you run out of weight to lose! Obviously this is a great problem to have, but it is still a huge issue that causes many people to backslide. Someone who will typically get stuck here will be the type of person that just can't get over the scale. They are now fit and healthy and they still weigh themselves all the time or are unable to find a new focus point that is non scale related. The person that pushes past this third pain point is someone who is able to become "special" in a different way.

At our studio we have large dry erase boards that hang high in the studio where everyone can see them. These are our weight loss club boards that go from 30lbs up to 200lbs of weight loss. There is tremendous momentum and energy that comes with charging up that board. All of our 100lb club members have felt that. People are clapping for you in class, we are blasting your transformation pics out on Facebook, and the momentum is huge! Then as you start to get close to being done with weight loss it is crucial that you are able to find that next set of goals, focus points, or things that motivate you. Many of our successful clients will start to look at physical goals at this point like running a 5K or obstacle course race or just improving their strength and body fat percentage. This can be a really awesome time in your transformation process if you can just get over the scale and get out of your own head about it! This is the big payoff where you get to test this new fit body that you have created. It should feel like you are out at recess every day that you get a chance to be physical and workout! One of our 100lb club members really nailed this transition and now she is a nationally ranked triathlete and heading to the world championships this year…..pretty darn cool!

So it all boils down to this: You need to be ready to tackle these three pain points. They WILL pop up. If you are brand new to working out and eating healthy you just need to be prepared. Think about each fork in the road and be ready to make the correct decision so you can move forward. If you have been at it for a while I want to challenge you to figure out where you fit within this timeline. How did you get through the pain points that you have crossed and which one is keeping you from moving forward?

- <u>Action Step:</u> Think about your past or current attempts at transforming your body. Make some notes on how far you have been able to travel along the Transformation Timeline. Do you tend to get stuck in the same zone? Are there any recurring issues that are keeping you from crossing to the next zone?

Understanding Past and Present Danger Zones

Ok, you are doing great so far! You are starting to see the big picture and look at your transformation in a new and exciting way. Now it is time to dig a little deeper into what has disrupted your transformation process in the past! I call these Danger Zones and they are a big deal! I see so many people waste their hard earned money by trying to do the same things over and over again and always failing with the same danger zones. They just assume that their next attempt will lead to different results and unfortunately they don't. I've had more than a few clients get into the "bootcamp zone" where they do our bootcamp for eight weeks, get great results, and then completely miss the point where they needed to start solidifying this new lifestyle. So six months later they repeat the process to re-lose the same weight. This isn't an efficient process! Using the Transformation Timeline as a guide is helpful with this. You need to analyze the three phases and think about where you have been stuck or if you landed in some danger zones. Once you have identified past danger zones you need to consider each one individually. With each danger zone think about what you are able to control and what was out of your control. Then come up with at least one action step that you can use to cross through that danger zone successfully the next time it happens.

My clients experience all different types of danger zones along their transformation process. One example I like to use is when people tend to cheat on their nutrition plan in the evenings after a long day of work. I think that this might be hitting home with some of you reading this! People have put in a full day of work and they just want to go home and decompress. The last thing on your mind is wanting to prepare a healthy meal so inevitably, more times than not, people hit the drive through window for something quick and easy. Let's think about what we can and cannot control in this situation. We can't have total control over the stressors at work. As we all know, that situation will vary on a day to day basis. We can control how easy it is to have access to quick healthy meals in the evenings. My favorite strategy to implement for this danger zone is to encourage clients to have two healthy food prep days per week. Usually one of those is a weekend where you can prepare healthy food in bulk. If you have a spouse and kids this can be an awesome family bonding moment as everyone pitches in to help prepare the food. Once the food is prepped you just package it up into containers so that you can heat it up in the evenings and you are good to go with minimal prep. I also like to add a second mid week meal prep day. My favorite strategy here is to use the crockpot. Just toss in some meat, veggies, water/broth, and spices and turn it on before you go to bed and when you wake up you have a few days worth of healthy dinners!

I want to repeat that your ability to identify, analyze, and strategize for your danger zones is really important because this is where a lot of time, money, and effort get wasted. By not repeating our past mistakes we can move through that transformation timeline effectively.

- Action Step: We are going to come back to your Danger Zones later on, but for now, start to make notes on the things that have tripped you up in the past. Think about one potential action step that you can take to prepare for each situation.

Establish Your WHY

So by now you know where you stand on the Transformation Timeline and what Danger Zones have caused you to fail in the past. The third thing that you need to consider before you start your transformation process is: "Why do I want to do this in the first place?".

Your WHY is a huge part of the third component that we have been preaching about so far. Having a motivating reason to take action means everything. I get excited when I sit down to talk to a client for the first time and they show some emotion. This means that they are emotionally invested in this process. I have many clients that shed tears of joy in our gym after a successful weigh in or after hitting a nice physical fitness accomplishment. One of my clients was motivated to start his journey because he felt that he was heading down a path where he wasn't going to have much quality time left to enjoy his grandkids. He still gets emotional when we talk about it. After dropping 80lbs he noticed that when his family members gave him hugs their arms would go all the way around him. He always gets emotional when recalling this. His WHY drove him to succeed no matter what.

Your WHY is very personal and it has to come from inside you. That is the tough part that many people struggle with. We have a lot of people that come to us because their doctor told them to lose some weight. This isn't a really strong WHY but we can enhance this. The WHY really needs to come from inside you and not by orders from the Doc. Most people are in this situation because their weight is impacting their health in a negative way. If we can make a mental connection with weight loss and increased quality of life, more time with loved ones, etc.....now we are building a stronger WHY. When I help people develop their WHY I like to ask them "What is going to keep you from hitting the snooze button for your 6am workout?" and then "What is going to keep you from hitting the snooze button *in six months from now*?".

With our local bootcamp program we used to really focus on people competing against each other and we've even given away money and prizes in the past. These motivators never led to long term success for the clients that were motivated by these tactics. Money, prizes, and competitions might motivate someone to get their foot in the door but it won't sustain them when it comes to solidifying a long term healthy lifestyle. You have to spend some time thinking about WHY you want to transform your life, your health, and your overall lifestyle and stay locked into that when times get tough! I like to say that your WHY has to be strong enough to out weigh all of your WHY NOT's. So if all the stuff hits the fan at once your WHY will keep you going anyway!

- <u>Action Step:</u> Make a list of your top five health/fitness goals. Now start asking the question "WHY?" and make notes until you get to the root of why you want to accomplish that goal. Now rank your goals from one to five in order of the strongest WHY.

Take the pressure off of yourself with this ONE simple mindset shift

With our local clients 90% of them start with what we call a Meltdown Bootcamp. These are immersive programs where we work on changing the first three components of the Amazing Results Formula (exercise, nutrition, and strategic thinking) all at once. The clients have a set plan to follow and we attempt to coach them through it and also hold them accountable to the plan at the same time. Sometimes we will see clients struggle with going through periods of being "ON the plan" or "OFF the plan" once their initial program wraps up. People put a lot of pressure on themselves over this concept and I want to provide a mindset shift that will allow you to take some of that pressure off.

With my one on one coaching clients we work on using a mindset of "As long as I have a plan, then I'm on the plan." It takes just a little bit of set up time, but once you have the plan in place it makes everything much easier. With our game planning we focus on mapping out four weeks at a time. We commit to a meal plan, a cheat bank, and an exercise regimen. I also make them commit to some sort of an automated reminder which will prompt them to set up their next four week plan. With this new mindset the only time that you are "off plan" is if you have no plan at all. Sometimes I have people ask me "When do I get to the point where I don't have to follow a plan?" and my answer is something along the lines of "When you are tired of making progress and you want to go back to your old body/health?". I feel like this is kind of like asking "When can I come to my job and just do whatever I feel like all day with no structure?" or "When can I start just writing down whatever I want for my taxes this year?".

Having some sort of a plan to follow actually makes everything much easier, more efficient, more effective, and overall less stressful. Not having a plan causes you to have to constantly tackle stressful situations in the moment and you may be ill equipped for those situations from the get go.

I want to go through a few typical scenarios and show you the difference between the old mindset of "OFF Plan/ON Plan" versus the new mindset of "I have a plan....so I'm on plan".

Scenario #1: I took two cheat meals today.

Old Mindset: I fell off the plan because I cheated. (This causes a sense of failure, loss of momentum, etc)

New Mindset: I have a cheat bank of six meals to use and these were two of them. I'm "on plan" because I have a plan and this was a part of it. (No pressure and no momentum loss).

Scenario #2: I had to miss my workout class today because I was sick.

Old Mindset: I fell off the plan because I didn't execute my goal for the day. (This causes a sense of failure, loss of momentum, etc)

New Mindset: I can take a class tomorrow instead or I can just count this as an extra rest day. I have a plan...so I'm ON Plan. (No pressure and no momentum loss)

I have picked up on the fact that clients put a lot of pressure on themselves to be perfect and they also tend to make our weigh in checkpoints these epic "make or break" moments. They get married to a number in their head that they *have to* achieve and then it causes a nervous breakdown if they are an ounce shy of that mark.

First we need to work on establishing the concept of "I'm on plan as long as I have a plan in place". Then we work on shifting the focus to the daily fundamentals that really matter. One bad habit that many people have is that they weigh themselves every day. We discourage this for a lot of reasons because you are constantly putting pressure on yourself. I spoke with one of my clients recently that admitted that she would adjust her diet daily based on what the scale said. I get the feeling that there may be more of you out there that do something similar. Once I get these clients to stop weighing themselves everyday we focus on the fundamentals that will make a difference. We ask daily questions like "Am I eating the right things according to my strategy that I have?" and "Am I meeting my weekly workout goals?". The pressure is taken off because we KNOW 100% that if we execute the fundamentals then good things will happen. The weigh ins are just a data point instead of some huge epic deal. Of course we celebrate victories on the scale as we get them, but our focus is on the execution of the plan and building those good habits. That is where the positive momentum happens. As these clients buy into what I'm telling them they notice an immediate pressure shift. I hear things like "I didn't have to stress about my weight all week long!"....and "That daily weigh in was the exact WRONG way to start every day!".

The way I see it is that we all only have so much energy to go around. Don't spend it on unnecessary stress. Instead channel that energy into powerfully positive habits that will help you reach your goals.

- <u>Action Step:</u> Think about how you can shift your focus point so that your transformation process is less stressful. Throughout this book we are going to help you formulate your transformation plan so that will definitely help! Make some notes on the things that stress you out about your transformation process and how you can make a shift in mindset or a tweak in the process to minimize that stress.

PART TWO:
GOING FROM GOAL SETTING
TO GOAL ACHIEVING

The Goal Achieving Process ™

So I want to make things easier for you, the reader, than I had it. It took me about ten years to fully develop my third component style of thinking and I want to help you learn to think this way in a much shorter time of course! I seem to be quite excellent at making mistakes, but I'm also pretty darn good at learning from those mistakes and figuring out better ways to do things. This Goal Achieving Process™ is no different. By now I hope that you realize that I am a product of this process and I've been able to fine tune things as I have lived according to these principles and applied them to my clients as well. I truly believe that if you follow this process, you will see a dramatic improvement with each goal that you have set for yourself. Spend some time with each success principle and really think about how it applies to you and your personal situation.

Success Principle #1: Find and Define Your Target

Let's say that we are playing a game of darts. If I were to blindfold myself, spin around in a circle for a few seconds, and then toss the dart there is a *chance* that it would randomly hit the bulls-eye of the dart board somewhere in the room. We all know that my probability of success greatly increases if I know where my target is and I can clearly see it in front of me.

So many people go out there and set random goals and then never do anything with them. They are chuckin' darts with a blindfold on! They are saying things like "I want to lose weight!", "I've got to fit into that dress by summer!", "I've got to get off these meds!" but it all ends with just a bunch of "holes in the wall" and nothing near a bulls-eye. Goal setting is just the first step in the process and unfortunately this is where many people get stuck and fail. We need to define what your bulls-eye is and where it is located. Then we will even go as far as to set a deadline to hit your bulls-eye just to add some extra focus and motivation.

Let's say that you and I were able to time travel to a place that is exactly six months from today's date. The good news is that you will have conquered the Goal Achieving Process™. Now looking back over the past six months what would have had to happen for you to be 100% pleased with your results? I think this is one of the BEST goal setting exercises you can do. Make a list of everything that you would assume that you would have accomplished if everything went 100% according to your plan. This is your chance to place your order and design a perfect six month period. The cool thing is that you can apply this process to any area of your life and I encourage you to do so! I want you to come up with at least five health and fitness goals that we can work with.

Now that we have some goals to work with we want to dig a little deeper. Let's say that one of your goals is to lose 25 lbs over the next six months. For a few days the thought of losing that 25 lbs will keep you motivated, but eventually that positive energy will start to fade and this is the area where most goals are put to rest. We have to make an emotional connection to your goal so that you become unstoppable.

Look over your list of goals and simply ask yourself "WHY?". Why do you want to do this? Then continue to ask yourself that question until you come up with an answer that creates emotion. So if your goal is to lose 25 lbs....WHY? Maybe your first answer is "because I want to have more energy"...ok...WHY? Then you figure out that you want more energy because you want to be able to keep up with your grand kids and THAT is the golden ticket my friends! When your diet becomes boring and those workouts become tough your WHY must be stronger than all of your WHY NOT's combined. The thought of losing 25 lbs won't always motivate you to get your butt out of bed at 5:30am for your boot camp class, but the thought of being able to enjoy your time with those grand kids will!

So once you have gone through this process with one of your goals go ahead and work through the rest of your list. You might find that some of the goals have a stronger emotional component and those are the ones that we need to focus in on. You may even decide to change up your list after doing this exercise and that is OK! The key is to find 3-5 goals that are going to mean the most to you and have the strongest WHY factor.

Now that you have solidified your WHY behind each of your goals it is time to sign a contract with the future YOU and create your own Lifestyle Rehabilitation Statement™. This will be your daily connection and focus point with your goals. Just setting goals and developing a WHY is not going to be enough. It is still too easy to lose focus and lose all of your momentum. A Lifestyle Rehabilitation Statement™ will allow you to focus in on what you want to accomplish and make baby steps towards those specific things each day. You will hold yourself accountable to these goals by reading the Lifestyle Rehabilitation Statement™ every single day.....twice per day!

Now remember my FIVE key rules for your Lifestyle Rehabilitation Statement™ that I mentioned earlier:

1. Everything has to be written with a positive focus.
2. Everything has to be written in the present tense as if it were already true.
3. You have to really try to FEEL IT as you read it.
4. There has to be a set deadline for completion. With this book I am encouraging at least six month deadline.
5. You have to commit to reading this statement *every damned day*, twice per day, until everything comes true or the deadline passed.

Here is a template that you can use as you form your own Lifestyle Rehabilitation Statement™. Remember that this may take a few tries and it is OK to edit this a little bit here and there as things develop.

The Lifestyle Rehabilitation Statement™ Template:

Today's date is (   ). I feel amazing because (   ). I'm excited about each day because (   ). I have gained so much positive momentum in the last six months because (   ). I am very proud of myself/family/friends because (   ).

Let's say that your top three goals look like this:

1. I will lose 25 lbs. (WHY? Because I want to be able to keep up with my grandkids and enjoy our time together)
2. I will run a half marathon. (WHY? Because I will feel empowered and unstoppable after doing this.)
3. I will throw away all my "fat clothes" and get a new wardrobe. (WHY? Because I will know that I'm never going back to that old *me*. This is the birth of the new and improved *me*.)

Your Lifestyle Rehabilitation Statement™ might look like this:

Today's date is (six months from today). I feel amazing because I have lost 25 lbs in the last six months. I can run and play with my grandkids and I even completed a half marathon. I'm excited about each day because I feel empowered with a new sense of self confidence. I have even thrown away all of my old clothes because they no longer fit. I am very proud of myself because I have been able to put "me" first so that I can both maximize my years and enjoy my time with the people that I love the most.

As you read this statement you have to really *feel* it. Imagine how you would look and feel if you were 25 lbs lighter. See yourself playing with your grandkids, running a half marathon, and wearing those new clothes. Feel that sense of being confident and empowered! It is important to really connect to this statement in this way for the same reason it is important to have that emotionally connected WHY behind each goal. The more that your body and mind are in sync the more likely it is that you will see daily opportunities to work towards your goals.

Imagine yourself in a long dark hallway. As you walk down the hallway you can't tell which doors are open and which ones are closed unless you feel around in the dark. Having a Lifestyle Rehabilitation Statement™ is like turning the light on so that you can see the opportunities that are open to you. You will start to see daily opportunities pop up that you would have missed otherwise because you weren't laser focused on those goals. For example you might notice an online coupon for a free personal training session or you might decide to skip the pizza that was brought in to work and eat a salad instead. As you capitalize on those daily opportunities you build momentum and start to feel unstoppable!

Success Principle #2: Get on the same side of the boulder

Transforming your body is one of the hardest things you will ever do because it takes hard work, discipline, and extreme focus. That goes for whether your goal is to lose 100lbs so that you can live a long and healthy life or to gain 10 lbs of muscle to look your best for summer vacation. Traveling from point A to point B in your own transformation process is going to take effort!

Imagine that you are standing at the base of a mountain and in front of you is a huge boulder. This represents your transformation process. All you have to do is put in a lot of focused hard work and effort to get that boulder to your goal at the top of the mountain. The great news is that you can recruit some people to help you push! Many people seek advice from health and wellness professionals when they decide to transform their bodies. You chose to pick up this book and read it which will allow me to help you push that boulder a bit. Whether you have a nutritionist, personal trainer, or you are in one of my online programs the absolute key is that we are both pushing in the same direction.

When you invest in some help from a health and fitness expert you are asking them to apply their knowledge and expertise to your unique situation. The problem is that many times people will not listen to the advice of these experts that they have hired. I remember some of my early personal training clients who I would design nutritional programs for and they would just completely ignore them and hit the buffet for lunch every day. I would kick their butt in our 60 minute training sessions and they would just counter balance that with poor food choices that didn't follow my guidelines at all.......and remember that was the advice they were paying for! We can push from opposite sides of the boulder and get some slow results, but why not join forces and propel you up that mountain *faster*! So from this point forward as you read this book I want you to think about whether or not you are pushing along side me or against me as you take action.

I use the word coachable a lot and the root of being coachable lies in being accountable. If you aren't being held accountable early on in your transformation process it is very likely that you will fail. So let's look at our mountain from a new perspective. I believe there are three steps to becoming self-accountable and you cannot skip steps because it won't work!

Step #1: Join a program that involves some type of accountability. This could be something like hiring a personal trainer, joining a bootcamp, or getting a group of friends together every Monday for a scheduled run. You have to join something where you are in a position where someone else could say "Hey...you aren't really following through on this!"....if you try to quit or back out. This is like standing in front of that boulder at the bottom of the mountain. You haven't done any pushing yet. You are just getting into position. Many people confuse this step with step #2 and that is a critical mistake.

Step #2: Allow someone to hold you accountable. Please take a second to notice the difference between this and Step #1. This is where you decide to actually start pushing alongside the person/people that are holding you accountable. So you are following the plan that your trainer gave you or you are showing up every week and kicking some butt with your run group. About half of the clients that my team and I have worked with will get slowed down in this area simply because it is hard to give up control. It could be an extremely grueling process like Bill had in my previous example or it could just be a couple of weeks as you figure things out and learn the system. An important focus point is to continuously work on getting better each day and follow the advice of your expert, trainer, or friends. If you hire a nutritionist and they point out a few errors that you have been making you have to make the adjustments that they request. That is being coachable and allowing someone else to hold you accountable. Anything less is just you pushing that boulder in the opposite direction. I honestly think that many health and fitness professionals and programs get a bad rap of "not working". It is more likely that the client is the one that isn't putting in the correct work and the "expert" just isn't asking them to give up control yet or at all. I'm just glad that I learned this lesson early on in my career. We always give our clients everything that we've got but sometimes you get a person that refuses to move from Step #1 to Step #2 in the accountability process and that is a major bummer!

Step #3: Become Self-Accountable. This is a great place to be but sometimes people put themselves here when they are actually still in Step #2. Many times we have people that finish an eight week bootcamp and they are flying high. The momentum is awesome and their confidence is soaring. This is a dangerous time for some that decide that they are now able to hold themselves accountable without any help. Most of the time these people have one or two good weeks and then they go right back to their old habits. Getting to the top of the mountain will take at least six months in my opinion. As you make your ascent up you have to collect as many Accountability Anchor Points ™ as possible. We will go more in depth into that principle in a minute, but the basic idea is that you need to build your support team as you go and keep that in place!

Here are some common traits of people that I have worked with personally that I consider to be self-accountable:

1. They don't have massive weight fluctuations. Most people reach a zone where their body is in the "sweet spot" where they feel and look healthy with a float range on their weight of a few pounds throughout a normal week. For example my bodyweight will vary during the week within a five to seven pound range depending on how sore I am, water retention, and carbohydrate/salt consumption.

2. They are goal driven and those goals aren't always about the numbers on the scale! At first when people have a lot of weight to lose they are all about the pounds. Then they reach their goal weight and an important transition point has to happen. You must be able to transition your goals to be more about fitness. Many clients look at their new body kind of like a brand new sports car and they want to see what they are capable of. I've seen our 100lb weight loss club members take on challenges like mud runs, triathlons, sky diving, and all kinds of other exciting things. As you work towards your physical goals, your weight and other health stats will continue to improve as a byproduct.

3. They are very consistent. They work off of a plan and have a regular regimen that they follow with their diet and exercise. They may change things up every once in a while but once the process is in place they really stick to it!

4. They are able to recognize a danger zone. Self-accountable people are very aware of what could potentially mess them up and they plan ahead to combat that type of a situation. They never fly blind into danger!

5. They are still willing to be coached as needed. I will go back to my example of Bill. We have some new programs and promotions every once in a while at our studio and if it makes sense Bill will plug in and learn some new tricks to add to his routine. If he feels like he needs a boost he will make the decision to get some coaching.

- Action Step: Now it is time for you to do a little bit of critical thinking. I want you to think about the different times that you have invested in a health and fitness program or product. Which step did you make it to in each situation? One of the hardest things for human beings to do is to "own it" and say that we messed something up. So really think about this concept. Did you just sign up and stand at the bottom of the mountain? Did you "kind of" follow the plan and push the boulder in the opposite direction as your coach, trainer, or friend? Think about where you are at right now with your current fitness plan and how you can start to propel yourself up that mountain and become self-accountable.

Success Principle #3: Develop Accountability Anchor Points

In the last success principle we talked about pushing that boulder up the huge mountain. With this success principle lets just pretend that we have to CLIMB up that mountain. As you climb it is critical to establish anchor points along the way. If you slip, the anchor point will keep you from falling all the way to the ground and starting over from the beginning.

There is nothing worse than losing a bunch of weight and then gaining it all back again. It isn't good for you mentally or physically and it is very hard to come back from. As my team and I help people along in their transformation process we help them establish accountability anchor points. It is critical that you collect as many accountability anchor points as possible as you transform. You never know when you will hit a rough patch. Life happens and you need to have a support system in place. If you don't, you run the risk of having to start at the bottom of that mountain again and it will look twice as big as before!

So let's talk about some of the different accountability anchor points that you can establish as you transform:

- Family/Friend/Co-workers: These people are on the front lines of your transformation process and they play a key role. These are the people that surround you when you are not in the health-friendly confines of your gym or fitness studio. You have to let these people know about your transformation and your goals. You also have to ask them to support you and hold you accountable. Sometimes people really luck out and have a great group of people around them, but most of the time there are a few in there that are just the opposite. It will almost seem like they are trying to sabotage you. Those are the people that you just can't worry about. Everyone deals with these types of people and you can handle it! Am I saying that you have to get rid of your friends and family members that don't support you??? No way! You just have to understand that everyone won't be on board at first and that is normal and you will have to step up and deal with it because YOU are worth the hassle.

- Regular fitness sessions: Having a regular fitness routine is an awesome accountability tool. You will develop relationships with the people that you are working out with and you should all help hold each other accountable. If one of your workout buddies disappears for a while you will need to check in on them and expect them to do the same for you. I am spoiled with the clients I have at our local facility. We have created a very unique culture where the peer to peer accountability is outstanding. People feed off of each other's momentum and the accountability connections just happen naturally. I realize that this isn't the norm across the country and you are going to have to put some work into it. You can start by getting a small group of supportive people (think about the friends, family, and co-workers from the previous note above) and take action together. Sign up for a series of personal training sessions, group classes, or a bootcamp and let the fun begin!

- Weigh Ins: At our studio we require our clients to come in every two weeks for a weigh in checkpoint. We hold them accountable but always provide positive feedback and support during these weigh in times. It is a good idea to have some kind of a results assessment as you transform. This could include weigh ins, measurements, body fat analysis, or a regimen of physical tests. We recommend that you do this every two weeks and not more often so that you have enough time to actually produce some noticeable results. Your weight will naturally fluctuate throughout the week depending on what you eat, drink, and how sore you are from your workouts. You should have a regular weigh in checkpoint day, time, and routine that you follow for the most consistent results. When you get your data just analyze it and see what you can do to make improvements over the next two weeks. As I have mentioned before…..don't freak out over your weight!

- Get some coaching: This is an area that my company specializes in. We take some of our most successful clients and train them in to be accountability mentors/coaches for new clients. This is a great accountability relationship because the new clients knows that their mentor has been in their shoes. When a client hires us for accountability coaching we take that very seriously. We will expect daily reports from the clients and we WILL chase you down for them! It is important that our clients really follow through with their plan and not fade off and lose momentum. I consider this the most effective form of accountability because all you have to do is follow the plan and send in your reports to your coach and you will get great results. It is all on you to get the job done, but you have an awesome mentor that has been through the same process successfully and they will do everything they can to help you reach your goals also. You will learn more about our specific coaching program later on in this book but if you just can't wait to check it out here is our website: www.TransformationCoach.Me. Many people take advantage of coaching through personal trainers, nutritionists, therapists, or life coaches as well. Having an expert on your team will always give you an accountability advantage.
- Journaling: Daily journaling in any form will be helpful in many ways. Even if you are just doing a simple written journal entry that no one else will ever see. The simple act of journaling will help keep you accountable on a daily basis. You could also step up your accountability by launching a blog or video journal to share with others. Just don't be one of those people like I mentioned in the intro

to this book..."Today I started my couch to 5K program...". I know that you won't, but I just wanted to remind you!

One important thing to note is that the goal is NOT to eventually be "free of any accountability" by becoming self accountable. We talked about this is Success Principle #2 and I want to re-emphasize it here. My definition of becoming self accountable is that you are at a point where you are not ever going to fall off the mountain and start back at the beginning. You won't gain all of your weight back or lose the results that you have achieved. You will still need to lean on your accountability anchor points often. You just have to find a way to mesh these into your new lifestyle that you are building.

- Action Step: Take a minute to analyze your current situation. How many accountability anchor points do you currently have? What would happen if things took a turn for the worse and the stress levels explode? Your WHY might be strong enough to power you through it, but then again it might not be. Who is going to be there to hold you accountable to your goals?

- Action Step: Make it a goal to be actively seeking accountability anchor points over the next few weeks. Try to get at least three solid ones in place. For example you could have a lunch time walking group that you do every Wednesday, sign up for personal training sessions once a week, and sit down with your spouse and tell them about your goals and how they can help you stick to the plan. The key, as always, is to stay actively engaged with this concept so that you don't fall off that mountain!

Success Principle #4: Take the fast track to build your momentum

Many times when people start their fitness journey they have a list of things that they want to improve upon or change. That is part of the goal setting process but we can't let this list dominate our thoughts because it can throw us off track quickly. With this success principle I want you to think about what you are already doing well. I believe that you already have 75% of what it takes to be successful and you just need a little help with that last 25% so that you can achieve your goals. If you are only focused on thinking about what you want to improve you are missing out on all of that positive momentum that you have already established. We all have to be sure to maximize our strengths in order to fast track our results.

This concept is particularly important when we are in a rut and struggling a bit. Here is an example that I see a lot with our local program. We have our weight loss nutritional plan set up in four phases with each phase being a little more strict than the previous one. Many times clients will be in a rut and struggling with sticking to the nutrition plan and they decide that they need to really buckle down and do phase four (the toughest one!). This is a recipe for disaster! What I recommend is that they pick the level that is the easiest for them to follow so that they have the best shot at success. If they are already struggling it doesn't make sense to take on the toughest challenge because if they fail it just adds to the downward spiral. So if you are struggling with establishing your fitness routine you shouldn't decide to set a goal to run 10 miles per day for the next two weeks if that is a huge challenge for you. Think about setting some goals that will allow you to get a few wins under your belt in order to re-establish your momentum like running a total of 10 miles per week.

Go through the questions below to help you figure out that 75% of what you are already doing well and what comes easy for you when it comes to health and fitness.

Fast Track List:

- What nutritional program is the easiest for you to follow and get results?
- If you are used to using a "cheat meal" or "free meal" system where you take days off from the nutrition plan….what has worked best for you in the past? You should pick a cheat schedule that allows you to feel like you are able to be social but also get great results. Finding balance with this is very important.
- Are you more likely to workout in the mornings or evenings? Weekends or Weekdays?
- What type of workouts do you enjoy the most: group fitness, machine cardio, strength training, personal training, online exercise, or exercise videos?
- Which friends or fitness buddies motivate you the most that you can connect with?
- What type of media can you plug into on a regular basis that pumps you up? (websites, tv shows, blogs, newsletters, podcasts, etc). Shameless plug: Check out my TransformationCoach.Me podcast……..it ROCKS!

Once you work your way through these questions you should have a nice outline for:

- A nutritional program
- A "cheat day" strategy
- A regular workout routine with specific types of workouts
- A group of fitness friends to keep you motivated and add accountability
- Some motivational media outlets to learn new tricks and keep you fired up

As you can see this is a really nice base! Some of you may be asking "What about that other 25%?". THAT is where having an expert to lean on comes into play. Having that expert (personal trainer, coach, nutritionist, etc) put the overall plan together is what allows you to hit your goals even faster. Once you know what you are already doing well and have a plan in place to hit your goals….you just have to follow the steps and you are well on your way to destroying your goals!

Success Principle #5: Know Your Enemy

We briefly touched on the topic of Danger Zones in part one of this book. Now it is time to go a little bit deeper. It is important to know what you are up against and have a plan of action in place for the worst case scenario. People that just "go with the flow" tend to hit a brick wall when their worst case scenario rears its ugly head and their transformation is in the tank. You are all going to invest a lot of time, money, and energy into your transformation so it would be silly to allow something to derail your transformation that could be prevented by a little bit of focused time each month to plan ahead.

I like to have our clients look at least one month in advance and identify any of these potential danger zones:

- Upcoming Holidays/birthdays
- Vacations/trips
- Business travel/meetings
- Stressful events
- Interactions with people that stress you out or can be a bad influence

Once you identify any potential danger zones for the month you need to come up with a plan of attack. This is a great time to look back at your work from Success Principle #4. Look at your areas of strength and apply those to help you come up with solutions for your potential danger zones. For example let's say that you are worried about your vacation that is coming up. You look back at your strengths and you love to workout in the morning and you tend to eat healthy as long as you start the day off right...BOOM...there is a great start to your plan of action for vacation. You should make sure that you get up before everyone else and knock out a quick workout and then start your day off with a healthy meal. This isn't rocket science and all it takes is a little bit of planning.

Another key point I stress to our clients is that the most important thing to worry about is what happens before and after the danger zone. You may blow your diet while on vacation but you can minimize the damage by preparing your body before you leave and having a plan in place for when you return. As I write this my family is preparing for a week long vacation to Disney World. I know this will be a danger zone because of limited food and fitness options. So I have spent some time thinking ahead so that I'm ready for this challenge. This preparation will allow me to actually enjoy my vacation more! To prepare for this trip I have been extra strict on my diet and I've been getting in extra workouts. You never want to enter a vacation on a fitness slump because that is a recipe for disaster! While we are on vacation I'm going to get in a 30 minute workout followed by 15-30 minutes of stretching and mobility work. We have access to what food will be available for our first meal of the day so I have that planned out as well. That way for the rest of the day I can just focus on having fun and making the best nutritional choices available throughout the day. Upon our return home I will snap right back into my strict nutrition and fitness routine.

With our clients I recommend that they sign up for a weigh in checkpoint right before and right after vacation for some added accountability. The idea is to spend just a little time planning ahead so that you don't add the stress of "failing on your diet/exercise regimen" to these already dangerous situations. Also don't put too much pressure on yourself. We all slip up every once in a while. The important thing is how you react to those slip ups because your momentum can shift quickly......for better or worse!

- Action Step: Look at your calendar for the next four weeks. Identify any potential danger zones that could disrupt your transformation process and come up with at least ONE action step that you can take to be prepared.

Success Principle #6: How to properly measure your success

Imagine that you are on a luxury cruise ship. You wave goodbye to the people from the back of the ship and then you decide to take a tour of the place as the ship prepares to launch. Fifteen minutes later you find yourself at the front of the ship and you are starting to wonder when the heck this ship is actually going to launch. You head to the back end to investigate and then you realize that you are miles and miles away from the shoreline and just didn't realize it.

As you go through your transformation process it is extremely important to remember where you started from. How did you feel? How did you look? Where were your confidence levels at? With the clients we work with we always have them do specific measurements and pictures from "Day One" as well. All of this "Day One" data is critical to your long term success so that you have a baseline that you can measure your progress against. Now before I describe this principle any further I want to share a story that explains a very common pitfall that you need to avoid.

One of our clients (we will call her "Cathy") had an ultimate weight loss goal of 40lbs. She got off to a very fast start hitting 10lbs, 20lbs, and 30lbs of weight loss very quickly. Once Cathy crossed that 30lb club she really started to put pressure on herself to hit that 40lb goal that she had set when she first started and things changed. Her weigh in success slowed down big time. She started seeing 1-2lbs instead of her normal 4-5lb drops. Then the weight loss completely stalled out and even reversed a little with some small weight gains. She was seeing these smaller numbers at each weigh in and the pressure mounted each time. She frequently said "That's ALL I lost!!!" and this added stress eventually ate away at her willpower and the cheats started to rear their ugly head. I knew that I needed to step in and decided that I would try something new with her next weigh in checkpoint. So the next time she came in I told her that we were only going to discuss her *total* results from the very beginning and not talk about what happens in each two week time span. I emphasized that she needed to celebrate her success and how far she has come from the *beginning*. So instead of thinking "I've ONLY lost 2 lbs!!!" she would say "WOW, I've lost a total of 32 lbs since I started!". This change of perspective made all the difference in the world. She had a much better attitude at her next weigh in checkpoint and I could tell that she was feeling less pressure already. Within a month she had not only hit the 40lb goal but she was already at 50lbs and tackling new challenges. She was free of the pressure and negativity that she was heaping onto herself!

It is very common to get trapped in this "measuring forward" mindset when you are close to a goal. We see this a lot when people approach certain milestones like weighing under 200lbs or under 300lbs for the first time. Once they start getting close people will put pressure on themselves and the results always slow down. I'm sure that the added stress does trigger some form of a hormonal reaction (increased cortisol) which can slow down progress, but I think the real problem lies with your decreased willpower. It has been scientifically proven that your willpower will fatigue just like a muscle and stress will fatigue your willpower more than anything else. What happens when we run out of willpower and we are on a diet? We crash and burn! So the vicious cycle goes on at each weigh in checkpoint with the stress building, willpower reducing, cheats increasing, and the results stalling out or reversing.

So the real key to Success Principle #6 is to always measure your results *from where you started*. It is a great thing to have big goals that you want to hit, but you have to realize that those big goals are a moving target. When Cathy hit her 40lbs goal she shifted her ultimate goal to 50lbs and then it shifted to doing a triathlon. Let your goals plow the road to success but *never* forget to look back and celebrate how far you have come since day one. If you catch yourself saying things like " I ONLY lost xyz!!!" or "That's IT???".....you need a shot of positivity and it is time to reflect on just how far you have come.

- Action Step: With our clients we use a tool called the Positive Progress Report where you write down different types of "WINS" that you have achieved since you started your transformation process.
  - Here are some examples:
    - What is my biggest mental WIN since I first started?
    - What is my biggest physical WIN since I first started?
    - What is my biggest nutritional WIN since I first started?
    - What is my biggest Friend/Family/Social WIN since I first started?

We recommend that you use this activity at least every eight weeks so that you can continue to let your goals motivate you and celebrate how much positive progress you have made since the day you started.

PART THREE:
FITNESS AND NUTRITION FUNDAMENTALS

Hopefully by now you are realizing how important the Third Component is. That being said, with this book we don't want to totally neglect the first two components of sound fitness and nutrition. I've included some notes in this section that should help you get off to a great start in those categories. You can also feel free to visit my website at www.TransformationCoach.Me and download my FREE Two Week Challenge packet which includes two weeks of our results producing nutrition plan and workouts.

Fitness Fundamentals:

There is so much information out there on different types of exercise that it can mentally wear you out before you even get started. I like to simplify things for the people that I get a chance to work with. Here are some key concepts to hone in on when you are thinking about a fitness game plan:

1. We need to MOVE and burn calories OFTEN. Working out once a week isn't going to get the job done.
2. We need to continuously adapt and make things a little bit tougher as our bodies adapt to the workouts. If you start out at level two on your elliptical machine it may be tough at first but as soon as you notice that things are getting

easier you MUST increase the intensity to get continued results.

3. We have to be as efficient with our fitness time as possible. You can't just go through the motions and talk on your cell phone while you do a leisurely stroll on the treadmill.

So to simplify these concepts even further you will need to consider exercise frequency, intensity, and efficiency when building your fitness routine.

The next step is to pick what types of exercise you are going to actually partake in. Again, we have about a million and a half options so here are a few things to consider:

1. Pick an exercise option that you are going to enjoy doing. Now I do use the word "enjoy" a little loosely here! One of my clients has a saying that goes as follows: "My most dreaded workout is the one that I'm heading in to do and my favorite workout is the one that I just finished!".....I love it! So the important thing to consider is how you feel AFTER you are done. Did you enjoy the process? Did you get a feeling of accomplishment?

2. Pick an exercise option that actually produces results! Remember that you aren't just handing out money! You have to expect results! You should walk out of your gym, studio, etc and feel like you have actually done something and the results should be measureable (scale, tape measurements, body fat %, pictures, etc).

3. Pick an exercise option that is efficient for you and your schedule. We are ALL busy....so that's not an excuse. We can all find pockets in our day to exercise. The key is to make the absolute most of that time. If

you only have 10 minutes a day you had better make it count. You won't get any results if you spend that 10 minutes sipping coffee and doing a few stretches.

A very common question that I get is "Should I start off doing group exercise or personal training?". My answer is "It depends!". My personal philosophy when putting a client through a transformation process is that I like to use group fitness for "cardio" or the part of the formula that produces a large calorie burn. I like to use personal training for fine tuning and working on things that a client couldn't get in a group setting. This is usually a very cost effective strategy.

If you are doing a personal training session and it is just a watered down (and much more expensive!) version of what you could get in a large group fitness class then you need to find a new personal trainer! With our program we usually use the personal training sessions for strength training. Everyone needs to do some form of strength training and this is also the area where many people tend to get injured if they are on their own and don't really have a clue what to do other than what they have read in a muscle magazine or seen on YouTube.

So for the average person that we work with we will have them focus on using group fitness for cardiovascular work and personal training for strength training work. Now there are a few variables to consider as well like your budget or if you tend to not enjoy the group fitness setting.

Nutritional Fundamentals:

With nutrition there are many options out there to choose from and there is bound to be a strategy that works for YOU. You just have to give the plan a chance to work by you *working the plan*. Here are a few fundamentals to consider as you form your nutritional plan:

1. Minimize the junk. If you eat unprocessed whole foods you are off to a great start. This should be the base of what you eat all the time. There is a lot of junk out there that is being marketed as "healthy". Remember that "organic" doesn't automatically mean "weight loss" or "healthy". If you smoked organic cigarettes they will still give you lung cancer. If you eat animal protein look for descriptions like "all natural", "hormone free", "free range", or "grass fed/grass finished". When you go grocery shopping stick to fresh products that are in their most natural unprocessed state like fruits, veggies, and nuts. If it didn't grow in the ground or in a tree try to avoid it. I'm pretty sure that I've never seen an Oreo Tree......just sayin!

2. Don't starve yourself. Think of eating as an act of fueling your body and your muscles for an active day. If you are hungry....see #1 above and eat clean. Weight loss is a combination of calorie intake and calorie burn. I would much rather see someone eat clean and be full so that they have the ability to give a little more with their workouts and burn off the required amount of calories to lose weight.

3. Don't put too much pressure on yourself to be perfect. Many times I will see people have one small slip up on their nutrition plan and it sends them into a huge downward spiral. With our clients we shoot for 80% efficiency with the plan. We feel like that kind of effort will allow the clients to get great results and still have room for small mistakes when "life happens".

What I learned from 365 days of perfect nutrition

I always try to choose to lead by example and I tend to take that to an extreme level. Many people struggle with taking too many cheat days, cheat meals, or just fade out on their nutrition too frequently. I got to a point where I felt like I needed to step up and show people that we all CAN be in total control over our nutrition no matter what is going on in our lives. To accomplish this I decided to stop taking cheat meals for 365 days in addition to avoiding any processed foods, sugar, caffeine, and artificial sweeteners.

Here are some of the basics of my battle plan:

- I broke up my nutritional program into two phases.
- Phase One would be a no carb and no cheat day/meal diet plan. The only "carbs" I ate were from green vegetables and nuts.
- In this phase I focused on protein, healthy fats, and veggies. I did allow myself to have grass fed beef to help me increase my healthy fat intake and overall calorie count as I was not trying to lose weight.
- I was going to stick to this phase until I felt like I was not performing well with my workouts and needed to add in some carbs.
- I ended up using this plan for the first 9 months of the program.
- Phase Two is the same as Phase One except I added in one healthy carb (fruit only) load day on Saturdays.
- So on Saturdays I was allowed to eat fruit with each meal.
- During this entire 365 day experiment I was 100% gluten free and 100% artificial sweetener free. Just by doing these two simple things I saw some amazing results with my energy levels, digestive tract health, quality of my sleep, and my workouts.

So what the heck was the point of this? I obviously enjoy eating healthy and reaping the benefits of that. I also enjoy being able to lead by example with our clients. The real driving force behind this 365 day experiment was that I really enjoy a good challenge. I feel like, as human beings we have to consistently push ourselves outside of our comfort zone and do things that are difficult. We *grow* and get better or we become weak and slowly die each day. I have always enjoyed doing things that other people would never do. When I was in college I competed in powerlifting and the squat was my weakest lift. I did some research and found a crazy Russian program that involved squatting almost every day of the week. All of my buddies and coaches said it was a bad idea but I was up for the challenge and decided to go for it full force. I couldn't walk correctly for about 6 weeks but when I tested my squat again I had added about 60lbs to my max and I was a lot mentally stronger as well.

So I attacked this nutritional challenge with the mindset that I was going to learn everything I could along the way and come out the other end better. I didn't weigh myself or track any stats because my goals weren't oriented towards those things. I can tell what I look like in the mirror when I weigh between 220lbs and 225lbs with low body fat and that was all the verification I needed during this time frame. I mainly wanted to focus on attacking each obstacle as it presented itself. I know that this is a huge issue for people that are trying to follow a nutritional plan. What to do when "life happens". A few times a year I will get a client email that sounds something like this:

"I need to put my program on pause because "XYZ" has happened. I'm under a lot of stress right now and something had to give and that is going to be my nutrition for now."

We are always there to support clients in this situation but when I read emails like this I always think "WHY?". Is eating poorly going to help you deal with stress? Aren't you going to have to eat anyway? Doesn't it take the exact same amount of time to eat something healthy as it does something that is not healthy?

So with this 365 day challenge I wanted to really analyze each life situation that popped up and learn from it. I had to figure out how to stay on my plan no matter what came my way. I kept track of some of the things that I had to learn how to deal with. Here is the summary list:

- Every single holiday and holiday parties
- What I learned: When you aren't focused on feeding your face during a holiday meal it helps you focus on the people. I had the best holiday season in recent memory because I was 100% focused on the experience of connecting with the people around me. This was truly awesome!

- My birthday, my son's birthday, everyone else's birthdays, and kid birthday parties.
- What I learned: In this category the most intense situation was taking my kid to other kid's birthday parties. Large groups of small humans STRESS ME OUT. That added stress factor combined with the seductive aroma of unlimited pizza was a test....at first. Then something happened. My four year old Henry was offered some pizza at one party and he said "No, but can I have a bowl of broccoli?"....NOW I SWEAR that I didn't put him up to this...the kid actually hates pizza! So that inspired me to stay strong and then it was no problem from then on.

- Sickness and injury
- What I learned: I push the limits pretty hard with my body and when I'm sick or injured I become a super wimp. I was only sick once, nearly puking during a Wednesday 6am class (Shout out to Coach Kerri for taking over mid class!). Once I was able to resume eating I just found some organic/all natural chicken and veggie soup. I've been dealing with back spasms for about the entire year also. Injuries can stress some people out but they really just motivate me to go into super recovery mode and be extra healthy to speed up the process.

- The health of friends and family
- What I learned: I had two pretty scary incidents of having to make visits to the emergency room. I sat and watched my father get his heart zapped back into rhythm on one occasion and the other was a great client and friend who had a seizure. Traumatic events like this can drive some people to eat due to the stress. Again, I had to look at the situation and consider "Will eating poorly in this situation help or hurt?". Do I need to spike my blood

sugar and go into a food coma?.....HELL NO! It is moments like these that your friends and family members need you to be sharp and at your best so eat accordingly.

- Travel (Chicago/Las Vegas)
- What I learned: I take a business trip to Chicago four times per year. This trip is easy because I know my surroundings, where I can score some food, and I can bring lots of supplies because I drive and have a fridge in my room. Vegas was a different animal altogether. This trip was during my last week of my challenge also so that made me extra motivated to dominate the experience! I just had to really plan each day and learn as much as possible. I had plenty of protein shakes, bars, almonds, jerky, etc to get me through as needed. Then I found places to eat where I could get veggies and meat.

- Work Stress
- What I learned: Any business owner will tell you how stressful it can be to run the show. Stuff happens all of the time that needs to be taken care of. I admit that I do have a huge advantage that my work environment is 100% healthy so that helps tremendously. I'm always motivated to be a product of the product so work stress is never really an obstacle to me staying on my nutritional plan.

- The birth of baby Hannah
- What I learned: This would have been a very easy time to break the rules and everyone would have understood, but I just couldn't go there! We lived in the hospital for four days and welcomed our new daughter to the world. I just had to make some trips back home or to the gym to pick up supplies because the hospital food was always questionable. I kept a cooler in our room and once again...I was able to focus on the experience....the WONDERFUL experience...instead of stress eating.

Here are a few takeaway thoughts:

1. The concept of food addiction is tricky. Food addiction is unlike any other addiction because you *have to eat* in order to survive. We can't just quit eating like we can with smoking, drugs, etc. After this experience I feel a little differently about the word "food addiction" though. I kind of feel like it is more of a combination of having cravings, some low willpower, low self esteem, and high stress more than being addicted to things like oreo cookies. The good news is that one thing can fix all of those things and that is POSITIVE MOMENTUM. The further I went along with no cheat days/meals the easier it got. To tell the truth...I kicked this challenge's ASS!

2. I know that some of you are starting to think about how you can apply all of this info to you. My advice would be to start small, make it low pressure, and include someone else. A great example would be to do a no cheat challenge with a family member or workout buddy for one month. Build from there once you have positive momentum established.

3. What happened on day 366? Protein and veggies baby! It would defeat the entire purpose of this challenge if I broke the rules on the first day after the challenge was done. That would be like going through rehab or alcoholics anonymous and then celebrating with a beer at the end.

Day 366 just meant that I had successfully completed what I set out to do and I was pretty damn proud of myself. Onward I go! (At the time of this book printing I'm crossing my TWO YEAR no-cheat anniversary....still going strong!).

Your nutrition, and really life in general, all come down to choices. When you come to an obstacle or a fork in the road will you choose to make the strong minded decision or the weak minded decision? With each strong decision made your willpower muscle builds and life gets easier. I challenge you all to challenge yourselves and push outside of your comfort zone every chance that you get. THAT my friends will enable you to truly LIVE and have amazing experiences along the way!

PART FOUR:
SAVE TIME, MONEY, AND EFFORT
BY AVOIDING COMMON MISTAKES

The Top Five Transformation Traps That You MUST Avoid

As human beings we are really good at sabotaging ourselves. That power is amplified when it comes to things that are difficult to do like transforming our bodies. We are experts in finding reasons why we can't do things or why our lack of success always seems to be someone else's fault. I've noticed a few "transformation traps" that seem to make people stumble during their transformation process.

Transformation Trap #1 Only having scale based goals: Most of our clients come in with some motivation to lose weight and that is totally normal. This particular transformation trap tends to rear it's ugly head a little further down the road. As people hit their weight loss goals they can quickly lose momentum and motivation if they don't have a new goal or anchor point to lock in on. To avoid this trap you should have a wide range of goals in categories like strength, endurance, body fat %, different measurements, energy level, activity level, mental state, etc. When people get towards the end of their weight loss journey and need to find a new focus point I like to use a real-estate analogy. I say "You started off with 100 acres of land and then you sell all 100 acres. How many acres do you have left to sell?"....They always say ZERO and then I remind them that they have run out of real-estate to sell so let's pick out a new focus point! One of my favorite success stories that deals with this point is Linda H. She hit her weight loss goal of 60lbs and then switched to a strength based goal of being able to deadlift her bodyweight. She accomplished that goal and now we are on to doing bodyweight pull-ups and dips and she is registered for her first obstacle course race. Did I mention that Linda is over 60 years old? Pretty awesome!

Transformation Trap #2 Weighing yourself every day: This is a very close relative of trap #1 above. People who are ultra focused on the scale tend to weigh themselves every day...sometimes multiple times a day. Sometimes I get emails that say things like: "Adam I'm FREAKING OUT....my scale says that I weight 0.75 lbs MORE than I did yesterday....what's wrong with me!!!!!! AAHHHH!". This is why we have a rule at my gym that you are only allowed to weigh yourself every two weeks and we recommend doing that with our official weigh in process at our studio. Your bodyweight will fluctuate all week long and throughout the day based on many factors including your soreness level, hydration, food consumption, salt intake, and many more. I'm all for measurement but I believe that you have to operate in a very strict and duplicatable environment to get accurate and comparable results. I weighed myself every day for a week for the purposes of this part of the book and I had a variance of 9 lbs throughout the week. That was actually the first time I had weighed myself in over a year by the way! Here's the real scoop with this transformation trap. If you weigh yourself every day the chances of freak out inducing weight fluctuations is very high. The more you stress over weight fluctuations the more that breaks down your willpower. That leads to stress eating and cheating on your nutrition plan. So stick to my recommendation of bi-weekly weigh ins in a controlled environment and stop freaking yourself out!

Transformation Trap #3 Going rogue in the first six months: With the first six months of any transformation process I always see a lot of opportunity. I've had several clients that have lost 100lbs or more right around that six month period. You can get a lot done....if you do it right. Sometimes people do a bootcamp or a fitness program for two to three months and then get over confident and decide to "go it alone" and be "self accountable". This usually ends in disastrous weight gain. Think of it this way, you have spent your entire life building up bad habits that have led you to the shape that you were in when you first started. Now you have momentum going but your new lifestyle isn't solidified yet and you still need to operate from a set plan, have a coach, and be accountable to someone else. Six months tends to be the sweet spot for our clients to achieve a higher level of self accountability and long term success. So stick to the game plan that is working! You don't need to prove anything by "going it alone."

Transformation Trap #4 Quitting because it starts to get tough: At our most recent bootcamp graduation I tried an experiment. I asked our bootcampers to think about how long they could hold a plank. I wanted them to focus in on deciding on their absolute maximum effort and what they could do. Then I asked them to add 30 seconds to that number and hit the ground and go for it. I told them to focus on what was actually going on with their body's strength and endurance levels and not just what they were feeling like "burning, shaking, etc". I'm happy to say that ALL of them hit their new goal and many of them doubled or even tripled their number. The moral of the story here is that people tend to pull back or quit just as something starts to get tough. This is often true whether we are talking about working out, diet, or even our relationships at home or in the workplace. The way I view struggle or difficulty is that it is usually a sign that I'm getting ready to hit a new level of progress. When you are experiencing some tough times it usually means you are just breaking through one of those pain points in the Transformation Timeline. This is the time to really focus in, work harder, and be even more disciplined! New results are right around the corner!

Transformation Trap #5 Measuring your results in the wrong direction: I know that we have already covered this, but I see this one mess more people up than all the other traps put together. The absolutely CRUCIAL aspect of this is that we let our ideal goals inspire us BUT we always measure from where we started. People get really messed up when they are ultra focused on that ideal goal (which tends to be a moving target by the way!). They are so dialed into that goal and "not being there yet" that they lose track of how much progress they have actually made. At each mini goal or measurement point you absolutely have to turn around and look back at where you started from and how far you have come. You've worked hard and you deserve to celebrate and be proud of yourself.

- Action Step: Are you stuck in one of these transformation traps? Take some time to honestly think about this and make a commitment to take at least one action step to escape each trap!

The ONE Decision That Can Make Or Break Your Transformation

The key concept I want to dive into here is the relationship between taking ownership and projection/blaming. When the "brown stuff" hits the fan are you looking to take control of the situation or point the finger of blame?

We all know at least one person in our lives that seems to always be full of drama. Bad things are always happening to them and they seem to somehow feed off of this! I lovingly call this type of person a "crap magnet". They are your friends, co-workers, or family members and you love them....but you don't want to get any of that on YOU. This is the type of person that tends to never accept responsibility for anything. Amounts of crap magnetism will vary from person to person. We've all had those moments when we decide to project our "crap" on other people and not accept any responsibility.

What I want to challenge you to do is the exact and polar opposite of being a projector or a "crap magnet". When a challenging situation arises I want you to search for a way to *own it* in some way. We can only control what we can control....I know....I just went Yoda on you! In any challenging or stressful situation think about what you can own. It is always very easy to blame other people and by doing that we are not really controlling what we can control. Other people are wild cards and they will do whatever they want. The sooner we realize that the better. Think about a situation in which you have recently placed some blame on someone else. Now think about controlling what you can control about that situation. What part can you take ownership over? If any of you are business owners you probably have had to fire someone at some point in time. That would be a great example to use for this activity. Usually the person has done something that has triggered the response of being fired. It is easy to place blame 100% on them. I've had to fire a few folks in my day and it is definitely not fun. As a boss and a leader of the organization I have to look at what I can control in the situation and how I can own it. Could I have trained them better? Could I have communicated more effectively? If you try this little exercise out you will find that your stress about the situation immediately decreases. Taking ownership will set you free where placing blame will only double the stress in any situation.

One key distinction to make is "taking ownership" versus "blaming yourself". When you take ownership over a situation you are making a positive move that will allow you to improve in the future. Blaming yourself has a much more negative impact and isn't productive. The real magic happens if a culture of ownership is produced where everyone is looking to own their part and improve from that experience.

So how does this all relate to your transformation process? Let me give you a couple of examples:

Example #1: The weigh in room is an emotional place. People are either going to be really excited or really disappointed. There isn't a lot of "in-between". When people ask me "What is the worst part of your job/career?" I will immediately respond with "weigh in room projection". This happens when a client hasn't been doing very well on their nutrition plan with lots of extra cheats. They know their weight will be up and they make a decision to project their stress onto me instead of taking ownership over the situation. I will have grown adults walk in there and say "This had better be good!" knowing that they have totally blown the diet. Then when they weigh in and see the weight is up they freak out on me about how hard they have been working, etc. They don't realize that I get reports from their coach about what they have been eating so I know exactly what is going on. This is a really tough situation to deal with and it happens more often than you would think! This is a case where people are going to project their lack of results as "the program didn't work for me"….when in reality they didn't take ownership and "work the program".

Example #2: We have a lot of clients that come to us that are in a situation where they are morbidly obese and they have to get the weight off to save their own lives. People don't become morbidly obese from just being lazy and eating junk all day. There are other things going on that have impacted them in a major way and food is the coping mechanism. The challenge here is to get these folks to "control what they can control" and not place the blame for their situation on their parents, spouse, boss, job, friends, etc. For these people to succeed they have to realize that they have to *own* their situation. They ultimately made the decision to put the food in their body and now they have to own it and take steps to improve their situation.

The basic idea here is that you have goals that you want to hit and we 100% know that life will throw some curve balls at you along the way. There is NEVER a totally perfect time to get fit, lose weight, get stronger, etc. When a challenge or stressful situation presents itself look for your opportunity to take ownership. What part of this situation can you control or make an impact on? Don't blame another person and don't blame yourself. Once you own your part, you are free to move forward towards your goal.

Here are a couple more examples of some of my clients that have stepped up in the face of adversity:

Example #1: We had a client that had a medical issue with one of her arms. She had to have more than one surgery where they actually broke her arm repeatedly to get it fixed......talk about a tough situation! This gal just owned it. She knew that the surgeries had to happen. She could not control that. She did know that she could control what she ate and she could find a way to still burn calories. By taking ownership over her situation she was able to lose over 50lbs by nailing her diet and doing all of her workouts one armed. She was in the studio working as hard as anyone else and it paid off. She didn't place any blame because she was too focused on controlling what she could control.

Example #2: This one happens all the time! We have lots of people that travel for business and have to attend conferences. This is an easy one to see the ownership vs projection relationship. We have had lots of people succeed in this situation by taking ownership. They call ahead to see what types of food will be provided. They bring some extra healthy snacks as emergency back up. Others will project and place blame where "They HAD to eat the food that was provided!". I've never seen a situation where someone forced you to eat unhealthy food. Maybe this happens in communist countries???? One of our accountability coaches and 40lb club members (shout out to Coach Jennie!) travels every week for work. She is a road warrior and her ownership over her situation is outstanding. She knows that she cannot control the fact that she is on the road five days a week so she has to deal with it if she wants to see positive results.

Here is one last insight: When you get into a tough situation and opt to take ownership, you will find that the other people involved will tend to do the same. Recently I had been chasing down a client that hadn't been around the studio in a while. When it came down to it I sent the "final attempt email" and I took ownership. I told them that I felt bad because I wanted so badly to motivate them to get back into action. I thought that they deserved good health and they hired me and my team to help them get there. I went on to say that I had failed to be able to motivate them to reignite their passion to improve their health. I ended by saying that I would be there to help out however I could. I just spoke from my heart and owned my part. I had sent several emails trying to get this person ramped back up to take action with NO response. After I took ownership over my part I think they were able to see the situation differently and they were back in our studio within a week! I think that many times clients go MIA and they assume that I blame them or are mad/ashamed of them. That is the furthest thing from the truth. I accept the responsibility to try and help you as much as possible and that includes pulling your butt off the couch to get you plugged back in. Sometimes I can do that and sometimes I cannot. Either way I own that situation and from that point the ball is in your court to decide to take action.

- Action Step: This may be the hardest action step so far. Please dedicate some focused time to think this one over because it is very important. Don't move on to the next part of the book until you have thought this one through! I want you to think about who/what you blame for where you are at in your transformation process. If you are obese...who do you feel is to blame? If you aren't getting the results you think you should be getting...who do you blame for that? Now think about controlling what you can control. What part can you take ownership of moving forward so that you can set yourself free of the blame game!

Understanding the *Results Per Dollar* concept

I think that the one thing that I see people worry about the most is back sliding with their results. They have invested time, money, and a lot of effort into a transformation and they don't want to lose what they have built up! As I have said before, I believe that the third component of the transformation process is where most people "fall off the wagon" and blow their hard earned results. It is important, however, to remember that you can't just sit at home and "think" away the pounds. You are going to have to get your hands dirty and sweat it out a bit. There are dozens of paths you can take when it comes to exercise and nutrition. Everyone will gravitate towards different opportunities depending on what you like and what gets the best results. As you try different things out it is important to be constantly looking for what is working versus what isn't working.

There are going to be two layers to this discussion with two questions for you to answer. Here is the first thing you have to ask yourself: *When it comes to my fitness/nutrition program am I just doing something or am I actually getting something done?*

Obviously there is a big difference between the two halves of that question and it can be a tough thing to assess for many reasons. As we have discussed before, one of the hardest things for human beings to do is take ownership over a perceived negative or "failure" situation. We naturally want to think that we are in the right and someone else is to blame. So I want you to just play along and pretend if you have to! We are going to step out of our own heads and analyze our situation. So ask yourself "Am I just doing something with my fitness and nutrition plan or am I getting something done?".

Another great way to phrase this question is, "Am I just taking some random action or am I actually seeing results?".

I think that any time you are investing your time, money, and effort into a fitness program you have to stay focused on the fact that you are not just buying "the program" you are actually making an investment in future results from that program.

Let that one soak in for a second because it is important to understand! I cut my teeth in a commercial gym for 10 years and it used to drive me crazy with the way people would shell out big bucks for multiple personal training sessions each week and they either looked the same (not a good thing) or worse over that ten year span. Now one clarification I want to make is that taking some sort of action is an amazing first step. You should 100% be proud of yourselves for taking that initial action. What I'm trying to hammer home here is that if you just keep doing the same thing with no results and no expectations of results then you are really just wasting a lot of time, money, and effort. That is the mental shift we are hoping to make here! I have a friend that I see once per quarter in a business group. He's from the east coast and he's had a personal trainer for the past five years. Every time I see him he tells me that he isn't happy with the trainer and hasn't seen any results yet. He's also paying his trainer $75 per hourly session! The reason he hasn't dumped his trainer yet is that they have become friends and he doesn't want to hurt his feelings. So he's doing three sessions per week at $75 per session. That comes to a grand total of $11,700 per year for a personal *friend.* This is insane and it happens ALL THE TIME. I would make a guess that a few of you have hired personal *friends*.

A great question to ask in this situation is "What are my results per dollar here?". If you get a $10 per month gym membership and gain 10 lbs of body fat over the course of a year that will equal very low Results Per Dollar or RPD. If you do a bootcamp for

$400 and lose 40lbs in eight weeks that is a very high RPD. Hopefully this is all starting to make some sense!

The next layer of this discussion has to deal with the following question: *"Who is to blame for the low results per dollar....me or the fitness professional/program?"*. Again....it is always easier to blame anyone but yourself so just for now...just for me....let's step outside of our own head and analyze this situation because this is the tougher of the two questions for sure.

Lets say that you hire a personal trainer. They set you up with a nutrition program and they run you through a workout twice per week. During the workouts they are super friendly and helpful. You give it 100% with the entire plan by following what they say. After six months of this you haven't seen any results. This is a situation where you need to change the program/professional you are using.

Now lets say that you hire a different personal trainer. They set you up with a nutrition program and they run you through a workout twice per week. You follow the nutrition program about half of the time and you don't really push it very hard during the workouts and sometimes you skip them. After six months of this you haven't seen any results. This is a situation where you need to get your head in the game and give the program an honest chance to work.

- Action Step: Ask yourself the question "When it comes to my fitness program am I just doing something or am I getting something done?" Make a list of the results you have accomplished so far. What do your results per dollar look like?
- Action Step: Ask yourself the question "Who is to blame for the low results per dollar....me or the fitness professional/program?"

PART FIVE:
FINDING YOUR HEALTHY LIFESTYLE BALANCE

I want to congratulate you for hanging in there and finishing off this book! Way to go! I realize that we have gone pretty deep with some intense issues that you probably aren't used to thinking about. A few days ago you thought fitness was just about eating right and working out and then I drop all of this heavy Third Component stuff on you! So I want you to take a second to pause, take a deep breath, and realize that this is going to take some time and effort to put together... but you can totally do this! You do need to have a game plan in place and everything you have read so far will help you get that done. You will need to tweak your plan often until you find your groove and then you will be in the zone!

As you begin to take action with everything we have set up so far I want you to keep one more big concept in mind. I call this "The Healthy Lifestyle Balance Finder" and it is a big deal(I think I've said that more than once by now!).

When people first kick off a body transformation process there is always an imbalance that motivates them to get started. Something in their lifestyle is causing them to be unhappy with their health/fitness. So the balance looks a little like this:

LIFESTYLE/health

This person may be eating too much junk food, not sleeping enough, or just not taking proper care of themselves in general. So they are motivated to do something about it. They may join a bootcamp, get a coach, or read a book with a nutrition system.

Now this next part is really important so tune in folks! The goal at this point is to stop the negative momentum that was caused by the imbalance and then we have to shift the momentum into a positive direction. This can only be achieved by creating a *short term* imbalance in the exact opposite direction like this:

HEALTH/lifestyle

There are going to have to be some sacrifices made so that we can get to this point in the process. You might have to give up some social time, some sleep time, and definitely some of your old nutrition habits. When I work with people we are going to ask them to give us at least eight weeks where they make their health and fitness a top priority. It is very easy for people to freak out during this phase. They will say things like "I can't maintain this!"

and they are exactly right. You have to realize that this is just one phase in the process and we are working on shifting that balance to the HEALTH side of the relationship. This is the most common area where people will give up because they don't understand the overall process. They are stuck with the old style of thinking that this is just the way it has to be forever. Now that you have been working on the concepts in this book, hopefully you are starting to develop a new way of thinking that involves the ability to see that this is just one critical step in the path to success. Ultimately, once great momentum is established and the poor health habits have been greatly reduced, we can start phase three of this process and start to find that healthy lifestyle balance:

Health/Lifestyle

In this part of the process we look to solidify the positive health habits and also ingrain these habits into a new and improved lifestyle that you are happy with. At this point you should be seeing awesome momentum with your health and feeling very satisfied with your overall lifestyle.

Here is a specific example of how this has worked with one of my private coaching clients. She got started because she was continuously on a yo-yo weight gain/loss pattern. Her food was way out of whack and her alcohol consumption was too high. We got started with a twelve week customized program that was pretty intense. I explained to her that we had to do this to shift her momentum into the correct direction. During this phase she was reduced to one cheat meal per week and any social alcohol consumption would count in that cheat meal category. She had to give me some more time in the gym, wake up earlier than she was used to, and she cut back on some of her social time with her friends and family. During this phase I had to keep reiterating that this was just a temporary, but very necessary phase, and the ultimate goal is finding that balance. As the results started to happen and momentum started to build we began to make our shift into the third part of this process. We added in some more variety to her nutrition program and required fewer hours in the gym. We also added a social alcohol cheat bank to use in addition to her other food based cheat bank. We had to communicate and work together to come up with that balance where I was happy with her continued positive progress with her health and she was happy with her new and improved lifestyle.

This is my goal with everyone I work with! I want to take you all on a transformation journey where you are ultimately able to look and feel the way you want to, and deserve to, along with living a fulfilling lifestyle that you feel great about. This balance is totally achievable but it is going to take a lot of hard work, as promised in the pages of this book. I always tell my clients that they can borrow some of my energy and momentum until they build up their own. I have been in your shoes and I can tell you that all of this hard work is 100% worth it because YOU are worth it my friend! Don't we all *deserve* have control over our health? Don't we all *deserve* to feel confident in how we look and feel?....Hell yes we do! It's your time to take ownership over your health and your lifestyle. Let's get after it!

ABOUT THE AUTHOR

Adam Schaeuble and his transformation team specialize in helping people that are interested in transforming their bodies, habits, and lifestyles. Adam helps his clients rehabilitate their lifestyles through specific strategic thinking concepts so that they can shorten their learning curve and experience greater results from any exercise or nutrition regimen. Adam is passionate about doing this because of his own experience with losing over 100lbs. He had a rock bottom moment in his mid twenties as he weighed 327lbs and was unhappy with where he was heading in life. He made a decision to start thinking strategically about his own health and this had such a profound impact on him that he became motivated to create specific systems to teach others what he had learned. Adam created the Meltdown Fat Loss Bootcamp in 2009 and over the next six years he was able to impact over 1,000 clients with over 35,000 LBS of weight loss results.....just in his home town of Bloomington, Indiana. In 2016 Adam launched his new website www.TransformationCoach.Me in order to expand his ability to make a positive impact. Adam obsessively pursues solutions to his client's danger zones so that they can reach new levels of personal achievement with their health and fitness.

TAKING ACTION WITH ADAM AND HIS TEAM

If you are interested in going deeper with the ideas discussed in this book please visit www.TransformationCoach.Me to see what programs and products are currently available. Be sure to join our newsletter list!

We also recommend that you follow us on Facebook (www.facebook.com/TransformationCoach.Me) for the most current program updates, free tips, and coaching videos with Adam and his team.

You can also subscribe to The TransformationCoach.Me podcast on iTunes or SoundCloud.

CLIENT TESTIMONIALS

"This has been super helpful for me putting the mental pieces of the puzzle together. I have had a lot going on in my personal life the last few months and this has really helped me pull my stuff together rather than flying off the handle and stress eating like I normally would! I would highly recommend it!"

Tobie R (100lb club member)

"Having a coach made all of the difference in my transformation. Your coach isn't just someone you email every night with your food intake. They're there to help you with every aspect of the program. Answer questions, provide suggestions and be there to cheer you on! So many times I've tried programs, and I may have had success for a while, but it was never long term. I was missing the most important part of any lifestyle change, someone to hold me accountable to it. I looked forward to getting that email from my coach every morning to fire me up for the next day! What made it even better was knowing that my coach had started as a client just like me."

Mandee F (100lb club member)

"I have been a client at Adam's studio for almost two years and I somehow managed to fall into a pattern of doing a bootcamp, doing well in bootcamp and then going back to my old ways. I couldn't figure out what normal life looked like. I knew that bootcamp was a time to "buckle down" and get things done, but what was I supposed to do after bootcamp?

When I heard through the grapevine that Adam was starting out these coaching calls I emailed him right away and asked to be on the roster.

So far I have completed 8 weeks of coaching calls with Adam and it has changed my outlook on how I view my fitness, what I consider my successes and how I handle the times when I stumble. There are times when I get on a call with Adam and say "I totally fell off the wagon last week and failed." After we finish the call Adam somehow has me believing that I succeeded.

In all seriousness, this has made a huge impact in my life overall. Adam has shown me ways to set goals for my weight loss and fitness that have little or nothing to do with a scale. These goals have taught me a new way of relating to my body and what I want to accomplish.

Adam has also provided me with reading recommendations and other tasks that have a positive impact on my overall happiness so that I feel secure in my mental strength to accomplish what I have set out to do.

I could go on and on about how much these calls have changed me. I don't think Adam even fully realizes what an impact he has had on me, and that he will have in the future on many others with these concepts.

More than anything, this has helped me find my new normal and how to make this lifestyle work with who I am as a person, without feeling that I am sacrificing or missing out."

Charlie S

"The benefits I experienced from having a coach worked like a well-oiled machine. I knew I had to report to my coach at the end of the day, so I had to keep track of what I ate. As a result of tracking what I ate, I was more aware of what I was putting in my body. Being more aware of what I was putting in my body led me to making better choices. Making better choices ultimately led to achieving the results I was working for. There were times that I would skip reporting for whatever reason (for the record, in hindsight, they were never good reasons!) and I definitely saw a correlation between that and my success. If I didn't intend to report, I felt like I could eat what I wanted because nobody had to know! But in the end, my body and the scale knew! The best part of my coaching experience was having the non-judgmental support, never feeling like I was being punished or ridiculed for slipping up. Instead, there was somebody there in my corner to get me back on track immediately. Not the next day, not the next week, but with the very next meal."

Nancy A

"The most helpful part about my interactions with my coach has been the constant support and suggestions for ways I could add variety to my diet and exercise, it helped me to stay focused. Knowing I had to report my actions and choices made me think twice about what I put in my mouth. The best part of the coaching experience has been the friendship and connection that we have developed through experiencing both the trials and triumphs together!"

Sheila H (70lb club member)

"I would say the most beneficial aspect of the daily coaching for me was just listening to them and knowing they had done or were doing the same things, both the workouts and nutrition, that I was doing. The accountability of the program is one of, if not the most important piece to me. The best part of the coaching has been the constant support and encouragement. The coaches make me want to keep on keeping on and also continue to learn and get better. Thanks so much for all you guys do everyday!"

Brad J (50lb club member)

www.ingramcontent.com/pod-product-compliance
Lightning Source LLC
Chambersburg PA
CBHW071215280526
45787CB00002B/686